INSULIN RESISTANCE DIET FOR BEGINNERS

A GUIDE TO RECLAIMING YOUR HEALTH

BY

OLIVER STONE

TABLE OF CONTENT

INTRODUCTION

Insulin resistance is a metabolic disorder in which cells in the body become less responsive to the effects of insulin. Insulin, which is produced by the pancreas, is essential for controlling blood sugar levels and allowing glucose to enter cells for energy. People with insulin resistance have cells that do not respond properly to insulin, resulting in higher blood sugar levels and increased insulin production.

Insulin resistance can be caused by a combination of genetic, lifestyle, and environmental factors. While genetics may make some people more prone to insulin resistance, lifestyle factors such as an unhealthy diet, lack of physical activity, obesity, and sedentary behavior are major contributors. Other risk factors include a family history of diabetes, certain medical conditions (e.g., polycystic ovary syndrome), and age.

Insulin resistance is strongly linked to the development of type 2 diabetes, as prolonged insulin resistance can eventually lead to the pancreas not being able to produce enough insulin to keep blood sugar levels normal. Additionally, insulin resistance is associated with various health complications, including cardiovascular disease, high blood pressure, dyslipidemia (abnormal lipid levels), obesity, and non-alcoholic fatty liver disease. It is important to understand the impact of insulin resistance on overall health in order to take proactive steps to manage and reduce its effects.

By gaining a comprehensive understanding of insulin resistance, its causes, and associated health risks, individuals can make informed decisions about their diet and lifestyle choices. With the right knowledge and strategies, it is possible to effectively manage insulin resistance and improve overall health and well-being.

CHAPTER ONE

THE SCIENCE BEHIND THE INSULIN RESISTANCE DIET

Grasping the role of insulin in the body is essential to understanding the science behind the insulin resistance diet. Insulin is a hormone produced by the pancreas that helps regulate blood sugar levels. When we consume carbohydrates, they are broken down into glucose, which enters the bloodstream. The pancreas then releases insulin, allowing cells in the body to take up glucose for energy or storage.

Carbohydrates have the most significant effect on blood sugar levels and insulin secretion. Simple carbohydrates, such as refined sugars and white flour products, are quickly digested, causing a rapid increase in blood glucose and insulin levels. Complex carbohydrates, found in whole grains, legumes, and vegetables, are digested more slowly, resulting in a gradual and steady release of glucose into the bloodstream. The glycemic index (GI) is a scale that ranks carbohydrates based on their effect on blood sugar levels. Low-GI foods produce a more gradual and controlled response, while high-GI foods cause a rapid increase in blood glucose and insulin levels.

High-fat diets, especially those rich in saturated and trans fats, have been associated with increased insulin resistance. On the other hand, lean proteins, such as poultry, fish, and legumes, can promote satiety, stabilize blood sugar levels, and support insulin sensitivity. Exercise is also a powerful tool for managing insulin resistance. It enhances insulin sensitivity, allowing cells to respond more effectively to insulin, and helps improve overall cardiovascular health, promote weight loss, and reduce inflammation.

By focusing on low-glycemic index carbohydrates, incorporating healthy fats and proteins, and engaging in regular exercise, individuals can optimize their diet and lifestyle to support insulin sensitivity, manage blood sugar levels, and improve overall health.

CHAPTER TWO

ASSESSING YOUR INSULIN RESISTANCE

Do you suspect you may have insulin resistance? It's important to recognize the common signs and symptoms that could indicate its presence. Not everyone with insulin resistance experiences noticeable symptoms, but some of the most common ones include elevated blood sugar levels, increased abdominal fat, acanthosis nigricans, fatigue and increased hunger, frequent urination, high blood pressure, and abnormal lipid levels. It's important to note that these signs and symptoms can also be indicative of other health conditions, so it's essential to consult with a healthcare professional for a proper diagnosis.

A healthcare professional can perform several diagnostic tests to assess insulin resistance. These tests can help determine the severity of insulin resistance and guide treatment decisions. Common tests include the Fasting Blood Glucose Test, Oral Glucose Tolerance Test (OGTT), Hemoglobin A1c (HbA1c) Test, Insulin Level Test, and Lipid Profile.

It's important to work closely with a healthcare professional to assess and manage insulin resistance. They can interpret test results, provide guidance on lifestyle modifications, and prescribe medications if necessary. A healthcare professional can also monitor progress over time and adjust treatment plans accordingly.

By understanding the signs and symptoms of insulin resistance and undergoing appropriate diagnostic tests, individuals can gain a clearer picture of their condition. This assessment serves as a foundation for developing a personalized treatment plan that focuses on managing insulin resistance through targeted dietary changes, exercise, and other lifestyle modifications.

CHAPTER THREE

CREATING YOUR INSULIN RESISTANCE DIET PLAN

Creating an insulin-resistance diet plan requires setting realistic goals that fit your individual needs and preferences. Think about your current health status, weight management goals, and dietary preferences. Achievable goals will help keep you motivated and ensure long-term success.

It's important to calculate your caloric needs when designing an effective insulin-resistance diet plan. Age, gender, weight, height, activity level, and goals (weight loss, maintenance, or gain) all factor into determining your caloric intake. A registered dietitian or online calculators can provide an estimate of your daily caloric needs.

The macronutrient balance in your diet is key to managing insulin resistance. Aim for a balanced approach that includes complex carbohydrates (fiber-rich, low-glycemic index carbohydrates like whole grains, legumes, and non-starchy vegetables), lean proteins (poultry, fish, tofu, legumes, and low-fat dairy products), healthy fats (avocados, nuts, seeds, olive oil, and fatty fish), and fiber (fruits, vegetables, whole grains, and legumes).

Meal planning and preparation are essential for maintaining an insulin-resistant diet. Plan your meals in advance, be mindful of portion sizes, cook at home, batch cook, establish regular meal times, and snack wisely (choose healthy snacks that combine protein, fiber, and healthy fats).

Fiber-rich foods, such as vegetables, fruits, whole grains, and legumes, should be a staple in an insulin resistance diet. Additionally, antioxidant-rich foods, such as berries, leafy greens, and colorful vegetables, can provide protection against inflammation and oxidative stress often associated with insulin resistance.

Staying hydrated is also important for managing insulin resistance. Drink adequate water throughout the day and limit sugary beverages, which can lead to blood sugar spikes.

By following these guidelines and personalizing your insulin-resistance diet plan, you can support better blood sugar control, enhance insulin sensitivity, and promote overall health and well-being. Don't forget to consult with a registered dietitian or healthcare professional for personalized guidance based on your specific needs and medical history.

CHAPTER FOUR

KEY FOODS TO INCLUDE IN YOUR DIET

If you're looking to manage insulin resistance, adding non-starchy vegetables to your diet is a great place to start. These veggies are low in carbs and calories, but high in fiber, vitamins, minerals, and antioxidants. Think leafy greens like spinach and kale, cruciferous veggies like broccoli and cauliflower, peppers, cucumbers, zucchini, asparagus, and mushrooms. Not only do they provide essential nutrients, but they also help regulate blood sugar levels and keep you feeling full.

In addition to non-starchy vegetables, lean proteins are also important for managing insulin resistance. Skinless poultry, fish like salmon and tuna, tofu, tempeh, beans, lentils, and low-fat dairy products are all great sources of lean protein. They help promote fullness, stabilize blood sugar levels, and support muscle maintenance.

Healthy fats are also key for an insulin resistance diet. Avocados, nuts like almonds and walnuts, seeds like chia and flax, olive oil, and fatty fish like salmon and sardines are all great sources of healthy fats. Just remember to practice moderation and portion control, as fats are calorie-dense.

Complex carbohydrates are also important for managing insulin resistance. Whole grains like quinoa, brown rice, and whole wheat, legumes like chickpeas and lentils, and certain fruits like berries, apples, and citrus fruits are all excellent choices. These carbs are digested more slowly, which helps regulate blood sugar levels.

Finally, incorporating superfoods known for their beneficial effects on insulin resistance can be advantageous. Berries, leafy greens, cinnamon, turmeric, and nuts and seeds are all great options.

Adding these to your diet can provide additional benefits in managing insulin resistance and promoting overall health.

By including these key foods in your insulin resistance diet, you can create a balanced and nutrient-rich eating plan that supports blood sugar control, enhances insulin sensitivity, and contributes to overall well-being. Don't forget to personalize your diet based on your specific dietary needs, preferences, and any guidance provided by a registered dietitian or healthcare professional.

CHAPTER FIVE

FOODS TO AVOID OR LIMIT

Managing insulin resistance requires careful consideration of what you eat, including avoiding or minimizing refined sugars and sweeteners. This includes sugary drinks, candy, desserts, pastries, and other foods with added sugars, as these can cause rapid spikes in blood sugar levels. Instead, opt for natural sweeteners like stevia, honey, or maple syrup in small amounts.

Processed foods are also a no-go, as they are often high in refined carbohydrates, unhealthy fats, and added sugars. This means avoiding packaged snacks, sugary cereals, processed meats, and pre-packaged meals. Trans fats and saturated fats should also be limited, as they can contribute to insulin resistance and increase the risk of cardiovascular disease. Sources of trans fats include fried foods, baked goods made with partially hydrogenated oils, and processed snacks, while saturated fats are found in fatty cuts of meat, high-fat dairy products, and tropical oils like coconut and palm oil.

High-glycemic index (GI) foods should also be avoided or limited, as they can cause rapid increases in blood sugar levels. Examples of high-GI foods include white bread, white rice, sugary cereals, potatoes, and processed snack foods. Instead, opt for lower-GI alternatives like whole grains, legumes, and non-starchy vegetables.

Alcohol consumption should also be moderated or avoided, as it can disrupt blood sugar regulation and contribute to insulin resistance. If you do choose to drink, do so in moderation and be mindful of its impact on your blood sugar levels.

By avoiding or limiting these foods in your diet, you can support better blood sugar control, improve insulin sensitivity, and reduce the risk of complications associated with insulin resistance. Focus on whole, unprocessed foods and prioritize nutrient-dense choices to optimize your insulin resistance diet. Consulting with a registered dietitian or healthcare professional can provide further guidance and personalized recommendations.

CHAPTER SIX

BREAKFAST IDEAS

1. Veggie Egg Scramble

Ingredients:

- 2 eggs
- A selection of non-starchy vegetables (such as spinach, bell peppers, mushrooms)
- Olive oil or cooking spray
- Salt and pepper to taste

Preparation:

1. Start by sautéing the vegetables in olive oil or cooking spray until they are tender.
2. In a separate bowl, whisk together the eggs with salt and pepper.
3. Pour the eggs over the cooked vegetables and scramble until everything is cooked through.
4. Serve hot.

2. Greek Yogurt Parfait

Ingredients:

- Plain Greek yogurt (unsweetened)
- A mix of berries (strawberries, blueberries, raspberries)
- Chopped nuts (almonds, walnuts)
- Cinnamon (optional)

Preparation:

1. In a bowl or glass, layer the Greek yogurt, mixed berries, and chopped nuts.
2. Sprinkle with a dash of cinnamon if desired.
3. You can enjoy it as is or add a bit of honey for extra sweetness (optional).

3. Overnight Chia Pudding

Ingredients:

- 2 tablespoons chia seeds
- 1 cup unsweetened almond milk (or any non-dairy milk)
- 1 tablespoon honey or stevia (optional)
- Sliced almonds or fresh berries for topping (optional)

Preparation:

1. In a jar or bowl, mix the chia seeds, almond milk, and sweetener (if using).
2. Stir everything together and then refrigerate overnight or for at least 4 hours until the chia seeds absorb the liquid and create a pudding-like consistency.
3. Top with sliced almonds or fresh berries before serving.

4. Oatmeal with Berries and Nuts

Ingredients:

- Half a cup of rolled oats
- One cup of water or unsweetened almond milk
- A mix of berries (blueberries, strawberries)
- Chopped nuts (almonds, walnuts)
- Cinnamon or vanilla extract (optional)

Preparation:

1. To make this delicious oatmeal, start by combining the oats and water/almond milk in a saucepan. Cook over medium heat until the oats are tender and the mixture thickens. If you'd like, you can add a bit of cinnamon or vanilla extract for extra flavor. Finally, top with mixed berries and chopped nuts before serving.

5. Vegetable Omelette

Ingredients:

- Two eggs
- Non-starchy vegetables (spinach, onions, tomatoes, bell peppers)
- Olive oil or cooking spray
- Salt and pepper to taste

Preparation:

1. To make a veggie omelette, start by whisking the eggs with salt and pepper in a bowl
2. Heat some olive oil or cooking spray in a skillet and sauté the vegetables until they're tender
3. Then, pour the whisked eggs over the vegetables and cook until the omelette sets
4. Finally, fold the omelette in half and cook for a few more minutes until it's fully cooked. Serve hot.

6. Avocado Toast

Ingredients:

- Whole grain bread (toasted)
- A ripe avocado
- Lemon juice

- Salt and pepper
- Optional toppings: sliced tomatoes, sprouts, or a poached egg

Preparation:

1. To make avocado toast, start by mashing the ripe avocado in a bowl and mixing it with a squeeze of lemon juice, salt, and pepper
2. Spread the avocado mixture onto the toasted whole-grain bread.
3. Finally, top with optional toppings if desired. Enjoy!

7. Smoothie Bowl

Ingredients:

- Frozen mixed berries
- Unsweetened almond milk or coconut milk
- Spinach or kale
- Chia seeds or flaxseeds
- Toppings: sliced almonds, coconut flakes, berries, or sugar-free granola

Preparation:

1. Blend together the frozen mixed berries, almond milk, spinach or kale, and chia or flaxseeds until smooth.
2. Pour the smoothie into a bowl and top with sliced almonds, coconut flakes, berries, or sugar-free granola.

8. Quinoa Breakfast Bowl

Ingredients:

- Cooked quinoa

- Unsweetened almond milk or coconut milk
- Chopped nuts (almonds, walnuts)
- Sliced bananas or berries
- Cinnamon or nutmeg (optional)

Preparation:

1. In a bowl, mix together the cooked quinoa and almond milk or coconut milk.
2. Top with chopped nuts, sliced bananas or berries, and a sprinkle of cinnamon or nutmeg if desired.

9. Cottage Cheese with Fruit

Ingredients:

- Low-fat cottage cheese
- Mixed fruits (such as berries, sliced peaches, or kiwi)
- Chopped nuts (almonds, walnuts)
- Cinnamon (optional)

Preparation:

1. In a bowl, combine the cottage cheese with mixed fruits and chopped nuts.
2. Sprinkle with cinnamon if desired.

10. Smoked Salmon and Avocado Wrap

Ingredients:

- Whole grain tortilla or wrap
- Smoked salmon
- Sliced avocado
- Fresh spinach leaves
- Greek yogurt or light cream cheese (optional)

Preparation:

1. Lay the tortilla or wrap flat and spread a thin layer of Greek yogurt or light cream cheese if desired.
2. Layer smoked salmon, sliced avocado, and fresh spinach leaves.
3. Roll up the tortilla or wrap tightly and slice it into smaller pieces if desired.

CHAPTER SEVEN

LUNCH AND DINNER RECIPES

1. Grilled Chicken Salad

Ingredients:

- Grilled chicken breast, sliced
- Mixed salad greens
- Cucumber, sliced
- Cherry tomatoes, halved
- Red onion, thinly sliced
- Olive oil and vinegar dressing (or lemon juice)
- Salt and pepper to taste

Preparation:

1. Gather all the ingredients for the salad in a large bowl
2. Add the salad greens, cucumber, cherry tomatoes, and red onion.
3. Slice the grilled chicken breast and add it to the mix
4. Drizzle with olive oil and vinegar dressing or lemon juice
5. Season with salt and pepper, and give it a good toss.

2. Baked Salmon with Roasted Vegetables

Ingredients:

- Salmon fillet
- Non-starchy vegetables (such as broccoli, bell peppers, zucchini)
- Olive oil
- Garlic powder, paprika, salt, and pepper

Preparation:

1. Preheat the oven to 400°F (200°C)
2. Place the salmon fillet on a baking sheet lined with parchment paper
3. Season the salmon with garlic powder, paprika, salt, and pepper
4. Toss the vegetables in olive oil, salt, and pepper, and spread them around the salmon.
5. Bake for about 15-20 minutes or until the salmon is cooked through and the vegetables are tender.

3. Turkey Lettuce Wraps

Ingredients:

- Ground turkey
- Butter lettuce leaves
- Garlic, minced
- Onion, diced
- Shredded carrots
- Hoisin sauce (look for a sugar-free version)
- Low-sodium soy sauce
- Sesame oil
- Salt and pepper to taste

Preparation:

1. Heat sesame oil in a skillet over medium heat.
2. Add the minced garlic and diced onion, and sauté until fragrant.
3. Throw in the ground turkey and cook until it's browned. Stir in the shredded carrots, hoisin sauce, and low-sodium soy sauce.
4. Cook for a few minutes, then season with salt and pepper.
5. Spoon the turkey mixture into lettuce leaves and serve as wraps.

4. Quinoa-Stuffed Chime Peppers

Ingredients:

- Ringer peppers (any tone)
- Cooked quinoa
- Ground turkey or lean ground hamburger
- Onion, diced
- Garlic, minced
- Spinach leaves, slashed
- Pureed tomatoes (search for a sans-sugar variant)
- Italian flavoring
- Salt and pepper to taste

Preparation:

1. Set the oven temperature to 375°F (190°C).
2. Remove the seeds from the bell peppers by cutting off the tops.
3. In a skillet, cook a ground turkey or lean ground meat with diced onion and minced garlic until sautéed.
4. Add cooked quinoa, tomato sauce, Italian seasoning, chopped spinach, and salt and pepper to taste.
5. Spoon the quinoa combination into the ringer peppers and spot them in a baking dish.
6. The bell peppers should be baked for 25 to 30 minutes, or until they are tender.

5. Pan-seared Vegetables with Shrimp

Ingredients:

- Shrimp, stripped and deveined
- Non-dull vegetables, (for example, broccoli, chime peppers, snap peas)
- Garlic, minced

- Ginger, ground
- Low-sodium soy sauce
- Sesame oil
- Salt and pepper to taste

Preparation:

- In a skillet or wok, heat sesame oil to a medium temperature.
- Add minced garlic and ground ginger, and sauté briefly until fragrant.
- Add shrimp and cook until pink and cooked through.
- Mix in non-boring vegetables and cook until fresh and delicate
- Sprinkle with low-sodium soy sauce, and season with salt and pepper
- Serve warm.

6. Chicken Breast with Broiled Brussels Fledglings

Ingredients:

- Chicken breast
- Brussels sprouts split
- Olive oil
- Garlic powder, paprika, salt, and pepper

Preparation:

- Preheat the stove to 400°F (200°C).
- Put the chicken bosom on a baking sheet fixed with material paper.
- Season the chicken bosom with garlic powder, paprika, salt, and pepper.
- Throw the divided Brussels sprouts in olive oil, salt, and pepper, and spread them around the chicken bosom.
- Heat for around 20-25 minutes or until the chicken is cooked through and the Brussels sprouts are fresh.

Ingredients

- Lentils (green or brown)
- Onion, diced
- Carrots, diced
- Celery, diced
- Garlic, minced
- Low-sodium vegetable stock
- Cumin, turmeric, paprika
- Salt and pepper to taste
- New lemon juice (discretionary)

Preparation:

- Under ice water, rinse the lentils.
- Sauté the diced onion, carrots, celery, and minced garlic in a large pot until soft.
- The cumin, turmeric, paprika, lentils, vegetable broth, and salt and pepper are now included.
- Heat to the point of boiling, then, at that point, diminish intensity and stew until the lentils are delicate (around 25-30 minutes).
- Change preparing if necessary.
- Get new lemon juice into the soup prior to serving, whenever wanted.

Ingredients:

- Spiralized or thinly sliced zucchini
- Grilled chicken breast
- sliced Tomato sauce (look for a sugar-free version)
- Olive oil

* Garlic
* Italian seasoning
* Salt and pepper to taste

Preparation:

* Olive oil should be heated in a skillet over medium heat.
* Add minced garlic and diced onion, and sauté until fragrant.
* Add spiralized or daintily cut zucchini to the skillet and cook until delicate.
* Add Italian seasoning, grilled chicken slices, tomato sauce, and salt and pepper to taste.
* Cook for a few more minutes to ensure that everything is thoroughly heated.
* Serve warm.

9. Heated Cod with Steamed Broccoli and Quinoa

Ingredients:

* quinoa cooked
* Olive oil
* Garlic powder, paprika, salt, and pepper
* Broccoli florets
* Cod fillet
* Lemon slices;

Preparation:

* Set the oven temperature to 200°C (400°F).
* Put the cod filet on a baking sheet fixed with material paper.
* Sprinkle with salt, pepper, garlic powder, olive oil, and paprika.
* Top with lemon cuts.
* Bake the cod for about 15 to 20 minutes, or until it is cooked through and easily flakes.

- Broccoli should be steamed until soft.
- The baked cod should be served with steamed broccoli on top of cooked quinoa.

10. Stir-Fry of Vegetables and Tofu

Ingredients:

- Cubed firm tofu
- Non-starchy vegetables like carrots, bell peppers, snap peas, and broccoli
- Minced garlic
- Low-sodium soy sauce
- Sesame oil
- Salt and pepper to taste

Preparation:

1. In a skillet or wok, heat sesame oil to a medium temperature.
2. Sauté the minced garlic until fragrant.
3. Cook the tofu cubes until just lightly browned.
4. Mix in non-boring vegetables and cook until fresh and delicate.
5. Sprinkle with salt and pepper and drizzle with low-sodium soy sauce.
6. Serve warm.

CHAPTER EIGHT

Finding healthy and satisfying snacks is an essential part of an insulin resistance diet. Here are some snack ideas that are low in refined sugars and high in fiber, protein, and healthy fats to help manage blood sugar levels and promote satiety.

Greek Yogurt with Berries:
For a delicious and nutritious snack, try plain Greek yogurt topped with a handful of fresh berries like strawberries, blueberries, or raspberries. Greek yogurt is packed with protein, while berries provide antioxidants and fiber.

Hard-Boiled Eggs:
Hard-boiled eggs are a great on-the-go snack that are high in protein. Boil a few eggs in advance and store them in the refrigerator for a quick and easy snack.

Celery Sticks with Almond Butter:
Celery sticks with a tablespoon of almond butter make for a crunchy and satisfying snack. Almond butter is full of healthy fats and protein.

Mixed Nuts:
Create a small handful of mixed nuts like almonds, walnuts, and cashews. Nuts are a great source of healthy fats, fiber, and protein. Just be mindful of portion sizes, as nuts are calorie-dense.

Veggie Sticks with Hummus:
Prepare snack-sized portions of sliced vegetables like carrots, cucumber, bell peppers, and celery. Pair them with a serving of hummus for added flavor and protein.

Cottage Cheese with Sliced Peaches:
Enjoy a serving of low-fat cottage cheese topped with sliced peaches. Cottage cheese is high in protein, while peaches provide natural sweetness and fiber.

Turkey or Chicken Lettuce Wraps:
Roll a few slices of lean turkey or chicken breast with lettuce leaves for a low-carb and protein-packed snack. Add some sliced cucumber or bell peppers for extra crunch.

Chia Pudding:
Make a batch of chia pudding by combining chia seeds with unsweetened almond milk or coconut milk. Let it sit in the refrigerator overnight to thicken. Add a dash of cinnamon or vanilla extract for extra flavor.

Edamame:
Enjoy a small bowl of steamed edamame for a plant-based snack that is rich in protein, fiber, and essential nutrients. Sprinkle with a pinch of sea salt for added taste.

Roasted Chickpeas:
Toss cooked chickpeas with olive oil, paprika, and a pinch of salt. Roast them in the oven until crispy for a crunchy and high-fiber snack.

It's important to listen to your body's hunger and fullness cues when snacking. Additionally, be mindful of portion sizes and select snacks that align with your overall dietary goals. These snack options can help keep you satisfied between meals while supporting your insulin resistance diet.

CHAPTER NINE

Satisfying your sweet tooth while following an insulin resistance diet doesn't have to be difficult. There are plenty of healthier dessert options that are lower in refined sugars and incorporate nutrient-dense ingredients.

Here are some delicious treats that can still provide a delightful end to a meal:

- **Fruit Salad:** Put together a colorful mix of fresh fruits like berries, melons, grapes, and citrus fruits. Add a squeeze of lemon or lime juice for extra flavor.
- **Greek Yogurt Parfait**: Layer plain Greek yogurt (unsweetened) with mixed berries, a sprinkle of chopped nuts, and a drizzle of honey or a few drops of stevia for a touch of sweetness.
- **Dark Chocolate-Covered Strawberries:** Dip fresh strawberries in melted dark chocolate with a high cocoa content (70% or more). Let them cool and harden before enjoying them. Dark chocolate contains antioxidants and less sugar compared to milk chocolate.
- **Baked Apples:** Core an apple and fill the center with a mixture of cinnamon, a sprinkle of oats or almond meal, and a drizzle of honey or maple syrup. Bake until tender and serve warm.
- **Chia Seed Pudding:** Combine chia seeds with unsweetened almond milk or coconut milk and a natural sweetener like stevia or a small amount of honey. Let it sit in the refrigerator to thicken, then top it with fresh berries or a sprinkle of unsweetened coconut flakes.
- **Frozen Yogurt Berries:** Dip fresh berries, such as strawberries or blueberries, in plain Greek yogurt and place

them on a baking sheet lined with parchment paper. Freeze until firm, then enjoy as a refreshing and nutritious dessert.

- **Banana "Nice" Cream:** Blend frozen bananas in a food processor until they reach a creamy, ice cream-like consistency. Add a splash of unsweetened almond milk or coconut milk if needed. Optional: Mix in a tablespoon of unsweetened cocoa powder or a handful of nuts for added flavor and texture.
- **Almond Butter Energy Balls**: Combine almond butter, rolled oats, chia seeds, and a natural sweetener like honey or dates in a food processor. Roll the mixture into small balls and refrigerate until firm. These make a convenient and satisfying treat.
- **Grilled Pineapple with Cinnamon:** Slice fresh pineapple into rings and sprinkle them with cinnamon. Grill until caramelized and serve warm. The natural sweetness of pineapple paired with the warmth of cinnamon creates a delightful dessert.
- **Coconut Chia Seed Popsicles**: Mix coconut milk, chia seeds, and a natural sweetener like stevia or maple syrup. Pour the mixture into popsicle molds and freeze until solid. These creamy popsicles provide a cooling and healthier dessert option.

No matter which of these treats you choose, remember to enjoy them in moderation and adjust the sweetness to your preference. By incorporating whole foods, minimizing refined sugars, and utilizing natural sweeteners, you can still indulge in healthier desserts while maintaining a balanced insulin-resistance diet.

CONCLUSION

In the end, following an insulin resistance diet is a great way to keep your blood sugar levels in check, support insulin sensitivity, and promote overall health. To create a personalized diet plan, it is important to understand the science behind insulin resistance and assess your individual needs. This includes knowing which foods to include and which to avoid or limit. Eating a variety of nutrient-dense ingredients such as non-starchy vegetables, lean proteins, healthy fats, and complex carbohydrates can help stabilize blood sugar levels and improve insulin response.

Moreover, it is essential to plan balanced meals and snacks, as well as to stay active. Opting for wholesome options like fresh fruits, Greek yogurt, lean meats, and whole grains will ensure a well-rounded and satisfying eating plan. Additionally, exploring healthier dessert alternatives allows for indulgence without compromising blood sugar control.

It is important to remember that it is best to work with healthcare professionals, such as registered dietitians or physicians, to get personalized guidance and support. With dedication, mindful food choices, and a comprehensive understanding of your body's needs, you can successfully manage insulin resistance and embark on a journey toward improved health and well-being.